PREGNANCY AND DIABETES

GORGEOUS ROSSY

TABLE OF CONTENT

DEFINITION OF DIABETES

Diabetes is a chronic medical condition characterized by elevated levels of glucose (sugar) in the blood. It occurs when the body either does not produce enough insulin (a hormone that regulates blood sugar) or cannot effectively use the insulin it produces. Insulin is responsible for facilitating the entry of glucose into cells to be used as energy. Without proper insulin function, glucose accumulates in the bloodstream, leading to high blood sugar levels.

There are different types of diabetes, including:

Type 1 diabetes: An autoimmune disease where the immune system mistakenly attacks and destroys the insulin-producing cells in the pancreas. People with type 1 diabetes require lifelong insulin injections or the use of an insulin pump to manage their blood sugar levels.

Type 2 diabetes: This is the most common form of diabetes, accounting for the majority of cases. It occurs when the body becomes resistant to the effects of insulin or does not produce enough insulin to meet the body's needs. Type 2 diabetes is often associated with lifestyle factors such as obesity, sedentary lifestyle, and poor dietary habits. It can sometimes be managed with lifestyle modifications, oral medications, or insulin therapy.

Gestational diabetes: This type of diabetes occurs during pregnancy and affects some women who did not have diabetes prior to becoming pregnant. Hormonal changes during pregnancy can lead to insulin resistance, resulting in high blood sugar levels. Gestational diabetes usually resolves after childbirth, but it increases the risk of developing type 2 diabetes later in life for both the mother and the child.

Causes of gestational diabetes

The exact cause of gestational diabetes is not fully understood, but it is believed to be a combination of hormonal, genetic, and lifestyle factors. During pregnancy, the placenta produces hormones that can interfere with the action of insulin, leading to insulin resistance. Here are some potential causes and risk factors associated with gestational diabetes:

Hormonal Changes: Hormonal changes that occur during pregnancy can affect the insulin action in the body. The placenta produces hormones like human placental lactogen, estrogen, progesterone, and cortisol, which can increase insulin resistance, resulting in elevated blood sugar levels.

Insulin Resistance: Insulin resistance refers to a condition in which the body's cells become less responsive to the effects of insulin. This occurs naturally during pregnancy to provide adequate glucose for the growing fetus. However, in some women, insulin resistance becomes more pronounced, leading to gestational diabetes.

Genetic Predisposition: Having a family history of diabetes, particularly a first-degree relative with type 2 diabetes, increases the risk of developing gestational diabetes. Genetic factors may contribute to the development of insulin resistance and impaired glucose metabolism during pregnancy.

Obesity or Excess Weight: Being overweight or obese before pregnancy is a significant risk factor for gestational diabetes. Excess weight can contribute to insulin resistance, making it more challenging for the body to maintain normal blood sugar levels during pregnancy.

Previous Gestational Diabetes: Women who have had gestational diabetes in a previous pregnancy are at a higher risk of developing the condition in subsequent pregnancies. They may have underlying predisposing factors that contribute to insulin resistance.

Polycystic Ovary Syndrome (PCOS): PCOS is a condition characterized by hormonal imbalances and insulin resistance. Women with PCOS have

an increased risk of developing gestational
diabetes due to their underlying insulin resistance.

Age: The risk of gestational diabetes tends to
increase with advancing maternal age. Women
who become pregnant after the age of 25 are more
likely to develop gestational diabetes.
Ethnicity: Certain ethnic groups, including Asian,
African, Hispanic, and Native American
populations, have a higher predisposition to
gestational diabetes compared to others.
It is important to note that while these factors
increase the risk of developing gestational
diabetes, not all women with these risk factors will
develop the condition. Additionally, some women
without these risk factors may still develop
gestational diabetes. Regular prenatal care and
screening are essential for early detection and
management of gestational diabetes during
pregnancy.

- *Importance of managing blood sugar levels during pregnancy*

Managing blood sugar levels during pregnancy is
of paramount importance for several reasons:

__Maternal Health__: Proper blood sugar control helps reduce the risk of complications for the mother. Uncontrolled diabetes during pregnancy can increase the chances of developing preeclampsia (high blood pressure), urinary tract infections, and ketoacidosis (a potentially life-threatening condition).

__Fetal Health__: High blood sugar levels in the mother can cross the placenta and expose the developing baby to excessive glucose. This can lead to macrosomia (large birth weight), which increases the risk of birth injuries during delivery. It can also raise the likelihood of the baby experiencing low blood sugar levels (hypoglycemia) after birth.

__Birth Defects__: Poorly controlled diabetes during early pregnancy can increase the risk of birth defects, particularly affecting the heart, brain, and spine. Proper blood sugar management before and during pregnancy can help reduce this risk.

__Preterm Birth__: Uncontrolled diabetes is associated with an increased risk of preterm labor, where the baby is born before 37 weeks of gestation. Premature babies may experience respiratory distress, feeding difficulties, and other health challenges.

Gestational Diabetes Management: Gestational diabetes, if not managed well, can result in complications for both the mother and the baby. By controlling blood sugar levels through dietary changes, regular exercise, and possibly medication, the risks associated with gestational diabetes can be minimized.

Long-Term Health: Poor blood sugar control during pregnancy can have long-lasting effects on both the mother and the child. Women with gestational diabetes have an increased risk of developing Type 2 diabetes later in life. Additionally, children exposed to high blood sugar levels in utero may have a higher risk of developing obesity and Type 2 diabetes in the future.

By effectively managing blood sugar levels, women with diabetes or gestational diabetes can significantly reduce the risks and complications associated with pregnancy. Regular monitoring, adherence to a healthy meal plan, appropriate physical activity, and medication adjustments (if necessary) are essential components of blood sugar management during pregnancy. Working closely with a healthcare team specialized in diabetes care during pregnancy is crucial to ensure the best outcomes for both the mother and the baby.

CHAPTER 2
• *Gestational Diabetes*

Gestational diabetes is a form of diabetes that occurs during pregnancy. It is characterized by high blood sugar levels that develop during pregnancy in women who previously did not have diabetes. The condition usually arises in the second or third trimester and resolves after childbirth.

Gestational diabetes occurs when the body does not produce enough insulin or is unable to effectively use the insulin it produces. Insulin is a hormone that regulates blood sugar levels. During pregnancy, the body goes through hormonal changes that can make it harder for insulin to work properly, leading to elevated blood sugar levels.

Risk factors for gestational diabetes include being overweight or obese, having a family history of diabetes, previous gestational diabetes in a previous pregnancy, having polycystic ovary syndrome (PCOS), and being older than 25. It is important to note that even women without these risk factors can develop gestational diabetes.

If left untreated or poorly managed, gestational diabetes can lead to complications for both the mother and the baby. The mother may experience high blood pressure (preeclampsia), a higher risk of requiring a cesarean section, and an increased likelihood of developing type 2 diabetes later in life. The baby may be at risk of excessive birth weight, low blood sugar (hypoglycemia) after birth, and an increased risk of developing obesity and type 2 diabetes later in life.

The diagnosis of gestational diabetes is usually made between the 24th and 28th week of pregnancy. Pregnant women may undergo a glucose challenge test, where they drink a sugary solution and have their blood sugar levels measured. If the results are abnormal, a follow-up glucose tolerance test may be conducted to confirm the diagnosis.

Treatment for gestational diabetes focuses on managing blood sugar levels through lifestyle changes. This includes following a healthy diet, monitoring blood sugar levels regularly, engaging in regular physical activity as recommended by a healthcare provider, and in some cases, taking insulin or other medication to control blood sugar levels.

Monitoring blood sugar levels is essential during pregnancy, and healthcare providers may recommend self-monitoring using a glucose meter. Regular prenatal check-ups are also important to assess the well-being of both the mother and the baby.

With proper management and treatment, most women with gestational diabetes are able to control their blood sugar levels and have a healthy pregnancy and delivery. After childbirth, blood sugar levels usually return to normal, but women who have had gestational diabetes have an increased risk of developing type 2 diabetes in the future. Therefore, it is important to continue monitoring blood sugar levels and maintaining a healthy lifestyle after pregnancy.

- ***Preexisting Diabetes and Pregnancy***

Preexisting diabetes refers to a condition in which a person already has diabetes before becoming pregnant. There are two main types of preexisting diabetes that can affect pregnancy: type 1 diabetes and type 2 diabetes.

Type 1 Diabetes and Pregnancy:
Type 1 diabetes is an autoimmune condition in which the body's immune system attacks and destroys the insulin-producing cells in the pancreas. Women with type 1 diabetes can have healthy pregnancies, but it requires careful management of blood sugar levels before and during pregnancy.

Preconception planning is crucial for women with type 1 diabetes. It involves working closely with healthcare providers to achieve optimal blood sugar control before getting pregnant. This helps reduce the risk of complications for both the mother and the baby.

During pregnancy, blood sugar levels need to be closely monitored and controlled. Insulin therapy is typically the primary method of managing blood sugar levels in pregnant women with type 1 diabetes. Regular prenatal check-ups are essential to monitor the well-being of both the mother and

the baby. Women with type 1 diabetes may have a
higher risk of certain complications during
pregnancy, such as preeclampsia, preterm birth,
and larger birth weight babies.

Type 2 Diabetes and Pregnancy:
Type 2 diabetes is a metabolic disorder
characterized by insulin resistance, in which the
body does not effectively use insulin. If a woman
has type 2 diabetes and becomes pregnant, it is
important to manage the condition to minimize the
risks to both the mother and the baby.

Preconception planning is also essential for
women with type 2 diabetes. Healthcare providers
may recommend lifestyle modifications, such as
adopting a healthy diet, engaging in regular
physical activity, and achieving a healthy weight
before becoming pregnant. In some cases,
medication or insulin therapy may be necessary to
control blood sugar levels.

During pregnancy, blood sugar levels need to be
closely monitored and controlled. Healthcare
providers may adjust the treatment plan to ensure
optimal blood sugar control. Regular prenatal

check-ups are important to monitor the well-being of both the mother and the baby. Women with type 2 diabetes may have an increased risk of complications during pregnancy, including preeclampsia, gestational diabetes, preterm birth, and larger birth weight babies.

It's important for women with preexisting diabetes to work closely with a healthcare team experienced in managing diabetes and pregnancy. They can provide guidance on blood sugar monitoring, medication management, nutrition, and lifestyle changes to ensure a smooth ride to motherhood.

• *Strategies for minimizing complications*

Minimizing complications in gestational diabetes involves a combination of strategies aimed at controlling blood sugar levels and promoting overall health during pregnancy. Here are some strategies that can help minimize complications:

Regular Blood Sugar Monitoring: Regularly monitoring blood sugar levels is crucial in managing gestational diabetes. It allows you to track your levels and make necessary adjustments to your diet, physical activity, or medication if needed. Follow your healthcare provider's recommendations for frequency and timing of blood sugar checks.

Healthy Eating Plan: Following a healthy eating plan is vital in managing blood sugar levels. Consult a registered dietitian or healthcare provider who specializes in gestational diabetes to create a meal plan tailored to your specific needs. Focus on consuming balanced meals that include whole grains, lean proteins, fruits, vegetables, and healthy fats. Avoid foods high in sugar and refined carbohydrates.

Regular Physical Activity: Engaging in regular physical activity can help regulate blood sugar levels and improve insulin sensitivity. Consult your healthcare provider to determine the appropriate type and amount of exercise suitable for your condition. Activities like walking, swimming, and prenatal yoga are generally safe for most pregnant women with gestational diabetes.

Medication or Insulin Therapy: If lifestyle modifications alone are not sufficient to control blood sugar levels, your healthcare provider may prescribe medication or insulin therapy. It is important to follow their instructions and take the prescribed medication as directed.

Regular Prenatal Care: Attend regular prenatal check-ups to monitor the progress of your pregnancy and assess the well-being of both you and your baby. These appointments allow your healthcare provider to make any necessary adjustments to your treatment plan and address any concerns or complications promptly.

Gestational Diabetes Education: Educate yourself about gestational diabetes, its management, and potential complications. Attend classes or programs specifically designed for women with gestational diabetes to learn about self-care, blood sugar monitoring techniques, and lifestyle modifications.

Support System: Seek support from your healthcare provider, family, and friends. They can provide emotional support and practical assistance in managing gestational diabetes.

Stress Management: High stress levels can impact blood sugar control. Find healthy ways to manage stress, such as practicing relaxation techniques, engaging in hobbies, or seeking counseling if needed.
Remember to follow your healthcare provider's advice and recommendations throughout your pregnancy. By closely managing your blood sugar levels, adopting a healthy lifestyle, and seeking appropriate medical care, you can minimize complications and promote a healthy pregnancy for both you and your baby.

CHAPTER 3

- ### *Blood Sugar Monitoring During Pregnancy*

Introduction:

Monitoring blood sugar levels is a critical aspect of managing gestational diabetes during pregnancy. Regular blood sugar monitoring allows you to track your glucose levels, make necessary adjustments to your treatment plan, and maintain optimal control. In this chapter, we will explore the importance of blood sugar monitoring during pregnancy and provide guidance on how to effectively monitor your levels.

The Importance of Blood Sugar Monitoring:

Assessing Glucose Control: Blood sugar monitoring provides valuable information about how well your body is processing glucose. By monitoring your levels, you can assess whether your current treatment plan, including diet, exercise, and medication, is effectively controlling your blood sugar.

Identifying Patterns and Triggers: Monitoring blood sugar levels helps identify patterns in your glucose fluctuations. You can track how your levels respond to different meals, exercise routines, stressors, and other factors. This information helps you make informed decisions about your diet, physical activity, and overall diabetes management.

Preventing Hypoglycemia and Hyperglycemia: Regular monitoring allows you to detect both low blood sugar (hypoglycemia) and high blood sugar (hyperglycemia) episodes promptly. Prompt identification of these fluctuations enables you to take appropriate actions to correct them, minimizing potential complications.
Blood Sugar Monitoring Techniques:

Self-Monitoring of Blood Glucose (SMBG): Self-monitoring involves using a glucose meter to measure your blood sugar levels at home. It requires a small sample of blood obtained by pricking your fingertip with a lancet. Follow these steps for accurate results:
a. Wash your hands with warm water and soap.
b. Insert a test strip into the glucose meter.

c. Prick your fingertip with a lancet device and apply the drop of blood to the test strip.
d. Wait for the glucose meter to display your blood sugar reading.
e. Record the result in a blood sugar log or on a smartphone app.

Continuous Glucose Monitoring (CGM): CGM systems use a small sensor placed under the skin to continuously measure glucose levels. The sensor transmits real-time data to a receiver or smartphone, providing a comprehensive view of your glucose trends. CGM systems may require calibration with SMBG readings for accuracy. Consult your healthcare provider to determine if CGM is suitable for you.

Frequency of Blood Sugar Monitoring:
Your healthcare provider will provide specific guidelines on how often to monitor your blood sugar levels. Generally, the frequency will depend on factors such as your overall glucose control, treatment plan, and individual needs. Common recommendations include:

Testing fasting blood sugar levels in the morning before breakfast.
Testing blood sugar levels one to two hours after starting meals (postprandial).
Testing blood sugar levels at bedtime.
Additional testing as advised by your healthcare provider in specific situations, such as during illness or changes in medication.

Interpreting and Utilizing Blood Sugar Results:
Understanding your blood sugar results is essential for effective diabetes management. Here are some considerations when interpreting and utilizing your blood sugar readings:

Target Ranges: Your healthcare provider will establish target blood sugar ranges for fasting and postprandial readings. Aim to keep your blood sugar levels within these targets to maintain optimal glucose control.

Collaborating with Your Healthcare Provider:
Share your blood sugar log or CGM data with your healthcare provider during regular check-ups. This information helps them evaluate your diabetes management, make necessary adjustments to

your treatment plan, and provide tailored recommendations.

Adjusting Your Treatment Plan: If you consistently experience high or low blood sugar levels, consult your healthcare provider before making any changes to your treatment plan. They can guide you in modifying your diet, exercise routine, or medication regimen to achieve better glucose control

CHAPTER 4
- ## *Insulin Therapy During Pregnancy*

Introduction:
Insulin therapy is a common treatment approach for managing gestational diabetes when lifestyle modifications alone are not sufficient to control blood sugar levels. In this chapter, we will explore the role of insulin therapy during pregnancy, including its benefits, administration methods, and considerations for its use.

Benefits of Insulin Therapy:
Insulin therapy plays a crucial role in maintaining optimal blood sugar control during pregnancy. Here are some benefits:

Blood Sugar Control: Insulin helps regulate blood sugar levels by facilitating the uptake of glucose from the bloodstream into cells. By achieving tight blood sugar control, insulin therapy reduces the risks associated with high blood sugar levels for both the mother and the baby.

Fetal Development: Insulin therapy helps ensure adequate glucose supply to the developing fetus, promoting proper growth and development.

Minimizing Complications: By effectively controlling blood sugar levels, insulin therapy helps reduce the risk of complications associated with gestational diabetes, such as preeclampsia, preterm birth, and macrosomia (excessive fetal growth).

Insulin Administration Methods:
Insulin can be administered using various methods during pregnancy. The choice of administration method depends on individual needs and preferences, as well as healthcare provider recommendations. Here are common methods:

Insulin Injections: Insulin injections involve using a syringe or insulin pen to inject insulin subcutaneously (under the skin). The injections are typically given in the fatty tissue of the abdomen, thigh, or upper arm. Short-acting, rapid-acting, intermediate-acting, and long-acting

insulin may be prescribed depending on blood
sugar control requirements.

Insulin Pump: An insulin pump is a small device
that delivers a continuous supply of insulin through
a small tube (catheter) placed under the skin. The
pump is programmed to deliver basal insulin
continuously and allows for additional bolus doses
before meals. Insulin pumps offer more flexibility in
insulin dosing and can help mimic the body's
natural insulin secretion patterns.

Considerations for Insulin Therapy Use:
When considering insulin therapy during
pregnancy, several factors should be taken into
account:

Individualized Treatment: Insulin therapy should
be individualized based on a woman's blood sugar
levels, insulin requirements, and overall health.
The type and dose of insulin may need to be
adjusted throughout pregnancy to maintain optimal
glucose control.

Regular Blood Sugar Monitoring: Blood sugar
levels should be monitored regularly to assess the

effectiveness of insulin therapy and make any necessary adjustments. Self-monitoring of blood glucose (SMBG) or continuous glucose monitoring (CGM) can provide valuable data for optimizing insulin dosing.

Healthcare Provider Guidance: Insulin therapy during pregnancy should be closely monitored and managed by a healthcare provider experienced in gestational diabetes management. Regular prenatal check-ups allow for adjustments to the treatment plan and ensure the well-being of both the mother and the baby.

Hypoglycemia Awareness: Insulin therapy increases the risk of hypoglycemia (low blood sugar). Pregnant women on insulin should be educated about recognizing and managing hypoglycemia. They should have access to glucose tablets or gel to treat low blood sugar episodes promptly.

Collaborative Approach: Open communication between the pregnant woman, healthcare provider, and diabetes care team is essential for successful insulin therapy. The woman should actively participate in her diabetes management, reporting any changes in blood sugar levels or concerns to her healthcare provider.

Conclusion:

Insulin therapy is an effective treatment option for managing gestational diabetes when lifestyle modifications alone are insufficient. With proper administration, regular blood sugar monitoring, and collaborative care, insulin therapy can help achieve optimal glucose control during pregnancy, reducing the risks associated with gestational diabetes and promoting a healthy pregnancy for both the mother and the baby

Types of insulin therapy

Insulin therapy is a common treatment for people with diabetes who have difficulty producing or effectively utilizing insulin. There are several types of insulin therapy available, which can be categorized based on their duration of action and timing. Here are the main types of insulin therapy:

Rapid-acting insulin: This type of insulin begins to work within 15 minutes after injection and reaches its peak effect in about 1 to 2 hours. It typically lasts for about 3 to 4 hours. Examples include insulin lispro, insulin aspart, and insulin glulisine. Rapid-acting insulin is often used to control blood sugar levels after meals or to correct high blood sugar levels.

Short-acting insulin: Also known as regular insulin, this type takes effect within 30 minutes to an hour after injection, with its peak effect occurring between 2 to 3 hours. It can last for approximately 3 to 6 hours. Short-acting insulin is commonly used before meals to control post-meal blood sugar levels.

Intermediate-acting insulin: Intermediate-acting insulin begins working within 1 to 2 hours after injection and reaches its peak effect in 4 to 8 hours. It can last for around 12 to 16 hours. Examples include neutral protamine Hagedorn (NPH) insulin and insulin zinc suspension. Intermediate-acting insulin is often used in combination with rapid- or short-acting insulin to provide both mealtime and basal (background) insulin coverage.

Long-acting insulin: This type of insulin starts working a few hours after injection and has a relatively steady effect over a longer duration, typically lasting up to 24 hours. Examples include insulin glargine, insulin detemir, and insulin degludec. Long-acting insulin provides basal insulin coverage throughout the day and helps maintain stable blood sugar levels between meals and overnight.

Premixed insulin: Premixed insulin formulations combine rapid- or short-acting insulin with intermediate-acting insulin in fixed ratios. They provide both mealtime and basal insulin coverage in a single injection. Premixed insulin is often prescribed for people who require a simple dosing regimen. Examples include 70/30 insulin (70% intermediate-acting insulin and 30% rapid-acting insulin) and 50/50 insulin.

The choice of insulin therapy depends on various factors such as an individual's blood sugar control needs, lifestyle, eating patterns, and personal preferences. It's important to work closely with a healthcare professional to determine the most suitable insulin regimen for each person's specific needs.

Considerations for managing insulin therapy during pregnancy

Managing insulin therapy during pregnancy requires careful consideration to ensure both maternal and fetal health. Here are some important considerations for managing insulin therapy during pregnancy:

Tight glycemic control: Maintaining tight blood sugar control is crucial during pregnancy to minimize the risk of complications for both the mother and the baby. High blood sugar levels can increase the risk of birth defects, preterm birth, preeclampsia, and other complications. Close monitoring of blood glucose levels and adjusting insulin doses accordingly is essential. Individualized insulin regimens: Insulin requirements can vary significantly during pregnancy, so it's important to tailor the insulin regimen to each individual's needs. Some women may require increased insulin doses, especially during the second and third trimesters, due to hormonal changes and increased insulin resistance. Regular monitoring and adjustments in consultation with a healthcare professional are necessary.

Meal planning: A balanced and consistent meal plan is important for managing blood sugar levels during pregnancy. It's advisable to work with a registered dietitian or diabetes educator to develop a meal plan that meets the nutritional needs of both the mother and the developing baby while keeping blood sugar levels stable. Insulin doses may need to be adjusted based on meal content and timing.

Self-monitoring of blood glucose: Regular self-monitoring of blood glucose levels is essential during pregnancy. It helps to identify trends, evaluate the effectiveness of insulin therapy, and make necessary adjustments. Healthcare providers may recommend more frequent monitoring, such as checking blood sugar before and after meals, as well as at bedtime.

Antenatal care and teamwork: Regular prenatal care is crucial for monitoring the health of both the mother and the baby. This includes regular check-ups, ultrasounds, and other screenings. A collaborative approach involving healthcare providers, including obstetricians, endocrinologists, diabetes educators, and dietitians, is important to ensure comprehensive care and management of insulin therapy.

Hypoglycemia management: The risk of hypoglycemia (low blood sugar) should be carefully managed during pregnancy. Women should be educated about the signs and symptoms of hypoglycemia and how to treat it promptly. It's important to have a plan in place for managing hypoglycemia and to carry a source of fast-acting glucose, such as glucose tablets or gel, at all times.

Education and support: Adequate education and support are crucial for pregnant women with diabetes. This includes understanding the importance of insulin therapy, self-monitoring of blood glucose, meal planning, exercise, and overall diabetes management during pregnancy. Diabetes educators, support groups, and online resources can provide valuable information and support.

Managing insulin therapy during pregnancy requires close monitoring, regular communication with healthcare providers, and adherence to the recommended treatment plan. It's essential to prioritize the health and well-being of both the mother and the developing baby throughout the pregnancy journey.

CHAPTER 6
● *Diet and Nutrition During Pregnancy*

Introduction:
Maintaining a healthy diet and adequate nutrition is crucial during pregnancy to support the growth and development of the baby and to ensure the mother's well-being. This chapter focuses on the key principles of diet and nutrition during pregnancy, including nutrient requirements, foods to emphasize, foods to limit or avoid, and practical tips for healthy eating.

Nutrient Requirements During Pregnancy:
a. Calories: Caloric intake should increase to support the growing needs of the fetus. An additional 300-500 calories per day is generally recommended.

b. Protein: Adequate protein intake is important for fetal growth and maternal tissue development.

Good sources include lean meats, poultry, fish, legumes, and dairy products.

c. *Folate*: Folate is crucial for preventing birth defects. Pregnant women should consume foods rich in folate, such as leafy greens, legumes, citrus fruits, and fortified grains.

d. *Iron*: Iron is needed to support increased blood volume and fetal development. Good sources include lean meats, poultry, fish, fortified grains, and leafy greens.

e. *Calcium*: Sufficient calcium intake is necessary for the baby's bone development. Dairy products, fortified plant-based milks, leafy greens, and tofu are good sources.

f. *Omega-3 fatty acids:* These essential fats play a role in fetal brain and eye development. Fish, walnuts, chia seeds, and flaxseeds are good sources.

Foods to Emphasize:

a. Fruits and vegetables: Aim for a variety of colorful fruits and vegetables, as they provide essential vitamins, minerals, and fiber.

b. *Whole grains*: Choose whole grains like whole wheat, brown rice, oats, and quinoa for added fiber and nutrients.

c. *Lean proteins*: Include lean meats, poultry, fish, legumes, and tofu for protein needs.

d. *Dairy or alternatives*: Opt for low-fat dairy products or fortified plant-based milks for calcium requirements.

e. *Healthy fats*: Incorporate sources of healthy fats like avocados, nuts, seeds, and olive oil.

Foods to Limit or Avoid:
a. *Certain fish*: Limit consumption of high-mercury fish like shark, swordfish, king mackerel, and tilefish. Choose low-mercury options like salmon, shrimp, and trout.

b. Raw or undercooked seafood, eggs, and meat: These can pose a risk of foodborne illnesses.

c. Unpasteurized dairy products: Avoid consuming unpasteurized milk, cheese, and other dairy products due to the risk of harmful bacteria.

d. Processed and high-sugar foods: Limit the intake of processed snacks, sugary drinks, and desserts.

Practical Tips for Healthy Eating During Pregnancy:
a. Eat regular meals and snacks to maintain stable blood sugar levels.
b. Stay hydrated by drinking plenty of water throughout the day.
c. Choose nutrient-dense foods to meet increased nutritional needs.
d. Practice proper food safety and hygiene, including washing fruits and vegetables thoroughly.
e. Listen to your body's hunger and fullness cues and eat when you're hungry.
f. Consider prenatal supplements as advised by your healthcare provider.

Conclusion:
Maintaining a well-balanced diet and proper nutrition during pregnancy is essential for the health and well-being of both the mother and the baby. By following the recommended guidelines, emphasizing nutrient-rich foods, and making informed choices, pregnant women can support a healthy pregnancy and optimize the development of their baby. Consulting with a healthcare provider or a registered dietitian can provide personalized guidance for individual dietary needs during pregnancy.

Recommended diet for women with diabetes during pregnancy

A well-controlled diet is crucial for women with diabetes during pregnancy to manage blood sugar levels and ensure the health of both the mother and the baby. Here are some general dietary recommendations for women with diabetes during pregnancy:

Consult with a healthcare team: It's important to work closely with a healthcare team that includes an obstetrician and a registered dietitian who specializes in gestational diabetes. They can provide personalized recommendations based on individual needs and help create a suitable meal plan.

Balanced meals: Focus on consuming balanced meals that include a combination of lean proteins, complex carbohydrates, and healthy fats. This can help maintain stable blood sugar levels throughout the day.

Carbohydrate counting: Carbohydrate counting is a common method used to manage blood sugar levels. It involves tracking the total grams of carbohydrates consumed in meals and snacks and adjusting insulin doses accordingly. A registered dietitian can provide guidance on carbohydrate counting and help create a carbohydrate-controlled meal plan.

Fiber-rich foods: Include fiber-rich foods in the diet, such as whole grains, legumes, fruits, and vegetables. Fiber slows down digestion and can help regulate blood sugar levels.

Portion control: Pay attention to portion sizes to prevent overeating. A registered dietitian can provide guidance on appropriate portion sizes for different food groups.

Regular meals and snacks: Aim for regular meal times and include healthy snacks between meals to maintain stable blood sugar levels and avoid extreme fluctuations.

Avoid sugary and processed foods: Minimize or avoid sugary and processed foods as they can cause rapid spikes in blood sugar levels. Opt for whole, unprocessed foods whenever possible.

Protein-rich foods: Include protein-rich foods in each meal and snack. Good sources of protein include lean meats, poultry, fish, eggs, legumes, and tofu.

Healthy fats: Incorporate healthy fats in moderation, such as avocados, nuts, seeds, and olive oil. They can help provide satiety and promote stable blood sugar levels.

Regular monitoring: Regularly monitor blood sugar levels as advised by the healthcare team. This can help identify any necessary adjustments to the meal plan or insulin regimen.

Hydration: Stay hydrated by drinking plenty of water throughout the day.
Remember, these recommendations are general, and it's important to consult with a healthcare team for personalized advice based on individual needs and medical history. The meal plan and dietary recommendations may vary depending on the severity of diabetes, medication use, and other individual factors.

CHAPTER 6

- **Exercise During Pregnancy**

Introduction:

Exercise during pregnancy offers numerous benefits for both the mother and the baby. This chapter focuses on the importance of exercise during pregnancy, the potential benefits, considerations, and safety guidelines for exercising while pregnant.

Benefits of Exercise During Pregnancy:

a. Improved cardiovascular health: Regular exercise helps strengthen the heart and improves cardiovascular endurance, which is beneficial during labor and delivery.

b. Increased energy levels: Engaging in physical activity can help combat pregnancy-related fatigue and boost energy levels.

c. Reduced pregnancy discomfort: Exercise can help alleviate common discomforts such as backaches, constipation, and swelling.

d. Better mood and mental well-being: Physical activity releases endorphins, which can help reduce stress, anxiety, and improve overall mood.

e. Weight management: Regular exercise can assist in maintaining a healthy weight gain during pregnancy.

f. Enhanced muscle tone and strength: Strengthening exercises can improve muscle tone, flexibility, and support proper posture.

Considerations for Exercising During Pregnancy:

a. Consult with healthcare provider: Before starting or continuing an exercise regimen, it's essential to consult with a healthcare provider to ensure exercise is safe based on individual circumstances.

b. Medical history and pregnancy complications: Certain medical conditions or pregnancy complications may require modifications or restrictions in exercise. These include preterm labor, hypertension, placenta previa, or a history of recurrent miscarriages, among others.

c. Type and intensity of exercise: Low-impact exercises such as walking, swimming, prenatal yoga, and stationary cycling are generally considered safe during pregnancy. High-impact activities or contact sports should be avoided.

d. Listen to your body: Pay attention to your body's cues and modify or stop activities if you experience dizziness, shortness of breath, pain, or contractions.

e. Proper nutrition and hydration: Maintain a well-balanced diet and stay hydrated before, during, and after exercise to support energy levels and prevent dehydration.

Safety Guidelines for Exercising During Pregnancy:

a. Warm-up and cool-down: Begin each exercise session with a warm-up and end with a cool-down to prepare and recover your body.

b. Wear appropriate clothing and footwear: Choose comfortable, breathable clothing and supportive footwear that accommodates the changes in your body.

c. Avoid overheating: Exercise in a well-ventilated area, avoid hot and humid environments, and stay hydrated to prevent overheating.

d. Pelvic floor exercises: Include pelvic floor exercises, such as Kegels, to strengthen the muscles that support the bladder, uterus, and bowels.

e. Modify exercises as pregnancy progresses: As the pregnancy advances, modify exercises to accommodate the changing body shape and avoid exercises that put pressure on the abdomen.

f. Pay attention to balance: Due to the shifting center of gravity during pregnancy, be cautious of activities that require good balance or involve a risk of falling.

Signs to Stop Exercising and Seek Medical Attention:

a. Vaginal bleeding
b. Persistent and severe headache
c. Chest pain or palpitations
d. Dizziness or faintness
e. Sudden swelling of the hands, face, or ankles
f. Leakage of fluid or contractions

Conclusion:
Exercise during pregnancy, when done safely and with appropriate guidelines, can provide numerous benefits for both the mother and the baby. It is important to consult with a healthcare provider before starting or continuing an exercise regimen to ensure it aligns with individual circumstances. By incorporating regular exercise, pregnant

women can improve their physical and mental well-being, manage pregnancy discomforts, and enhance their overall health and fitness.

The types and frequency of exercise during pregnancy

The types and frequency of exercise during pregnancy may vary depending on individual circumstances and medical history. However, the following are some recommended types of exercise and general guidelines for frequency during pregnancy:

Aerobic exercises:
Walking: Walking is a low-impact exercise that can be easily incorporated into daily routine. Aim for at least 30 minutes of brisk walking most days of the week.

Swimming: Swimming and water aerobics are excellent choices as they provide buoyancy and minimize strain on joints. Engage in swimming or water-based activities for 150 minutes per week. Prenatal yoga and stretching:

Prenatal yoga: Prenatal yoga classes or guided prenatal yoga videos can help improve flexibility, promote relaxation, and strengthen muscles. Aim for one to three sessions per week.

Stretching: Gentle stretching exercises can help alleviate muscle tension and improve flexibility. Incorporate stretching into your routine on a daily basis.

Strength training:
Modified strength training: Engage in strength training exercises that target major muscle groups using light to moderate weights or resistance bands. Focus on proper form and avoid heavy weights or exercises that put excessive strain on the abdominal area.
Aim for two to three sessions of strength training per week, allowing at least 48 hours of rest between sessions.

Pelvic floor exercises:

Kegel exercises: Pelvic floor exercises, known as Kegels, can help strengthen the muscles that

support the bladder, uterus, and bowels. Perform Kegel exercises regularly, aiming for several sets of 10 repetitions throughout the day.
General exercise guidelines during pregnancy:

Warm-up and cool-down: Always begin each exercise session with a warm-up to prepare your body and end with a cool-down to gradually reduce your heart rate.

Listen to your body: Pay attention to how you feel during exercise. If you experience any discomfort, dizziness, or pain, modify or stop the activity and consult your healthcare provider.

Stay hydrated: Drink plenty of water before, during, and after exercise to prevent dehydration. Wear appropriate clothing and footwear: Choose comfortable, breathable clothing and supportive footwear that accommodates the changes in your body.

Modify exercises as pregnancy progresses: As your pregnancy advances, modify exercises to accommodate the changing body shape and avoid exercises that put pressure on the abdomen.

Consult with a healthcare provider: Always consult with your healthcare provider before starting or continuing an exercise regimen to ensure it is safe for you and your baby. Remember, these recommendations are general and may not be suitable for everyone. It is important to consult with your healthcare provider or a prenatal exercise specialist to receive personalized recommendations based on your specific needs and circumstances.

CHAPTER 7
Complications of Diabetes During Pregnancy

Introduction:
Diabetes during pregnancy can present various challenges and potential complications for both the mother and the baby. This chapter focuses on the complications associated with diabetes during pregnancy, their potential risks, and the importance of proper management and medical care.

Gestational Diabetes Complications:
a. Macrosomia: Uncontrolled gestational diabetes can lead to excessive fetal growth, resulting in macrosomia (a large baby), which can increase the risk of complications during delivery.

b. Birth injuries: A large baby may increase the likelihood of birth injuries, such as shoulder dystocia (when the baby's shoulder becomes stuck during delivery).

c. Preterm birth: Women with gestational diabetes have a higher risk of delivering prematurely.

d. Respiratory distress syndrome (RDS): Babies born to mothers with poorly controlled gestational diabetes may be at risk of developing RDS, a condition characterized by breathing difficulties.

e. Hypoglycemia: Newborns of mothers with gestational diabetes may experience low blood sugar levels after birth.

f. Increased risk of developing type 2 diabetes: Both the mother and the child have an increased risk of developing type 2 diabetes later in life.

Preexisting Diabetes Complications:

a. Preeclampsia: Women with preexisting diabetes have a higher risk of developing preeclampsia, a condition characterized by high blood pressure and organ damage.
b. Diabetic ketoacidosis (DKA): DKA is a severe complication of diabetes that can occur during

pregnancy if blood sugar levels become dangerously high.

c. Congenital disabilities: Poorly controlled diabetes during early pregnancy increases the risk of congenital disabilities in the baby, particularly affecting the heart, spine, and kidneys.

d. Fetal growth problems: Poorly controlled diabetes can affect the baby's growth, leading to intrauterine growth restriction (IUGR).

e. Stillbirth: Poorly controlled diabetes increases the risk of stillbirth.

Management and Prevention:

a. Regular medical care: Seek regular prenatal care and work closely with a healthcare team that includes an obstetrician and an endocrinologist or diabetes specialist.

b. Blood sugar monitoring: Regularly monitor blood sugar levels as advised by the healthcare team and follow their recommended target ranges.

c. Medication and insulin therapy: If needed, follow the prescribed medication and insulin therapy regimen as directed by the healthcare team to maintain optimal blood sugar control.

d. Healthy diet and physical activity: Follow a balanced diet and engage in regular physical activity as recommended by the healthcare team to support blood sugar management.

e. Blood pressure control: Monitor and control blood pressure levels to reduce the risk of complications such as preeclampsia.

f. Education and support: Seek diabetes education and support services to learn about managing diabetes during pregnancy, including meal planning, self-care, and coping strategies.

Conclusion:
Diabetes during pregnancy, whether gestational or preexisting, requires careful management and medical attention to minimize the risks and complications for both the mother and the baby. By receiving proper prenatal care, closely monitoring blood sugar levels, following a healthy lifestyle,

and working closely with a healthcare team, women with diabetes can increase the likelihood of a healthy pregnancy and delivery. It is crucial to stay informed, educated, and proactive in managing diabetes during pregnancy to ensure the best possible outcomes for both the mother and the baby.

CHAPTER 8

• *Recommended care and monitoring for women with diabetes after delivery*

After delivery, women with diabetes require ongoing care and monitoring to ensure their well-being and manage their diabetes effectively. Here are some recommended care and monitoring measures for women with diabetes after delivery:

Postpartum medical check-up: Schedule a postpartum visit with your healthcare provider within 6 weeks after delivery. This visit allows your healthcare provider to assess your overall health, monitor your blood sugar levels, and address any concerns or questions you may have.

Blood sugar monitoring: Continue monitoring your blood sugar levels as recommended by your healthcare provider. This may involve regular self-monitoring of blood glucose using a glucose meter. Tracking your blood sugar levels can help identify any changes or fluctuations that require adjustment in your treatment plan.

Medication and insulin management: If you were taking medication or insulin during pregnancy, your healthcare provider will guide you on adjusting or discontinuing the medication postpartum. Follow their instructions and continue any prescribed medication or insulin regimen as directed.

Breastfeeding considerations: If you choose to breastfeed, consult with your healthcare provider and a lactation specialist to ensure that your diabetes management aligns with your breastfeeding goals. Managing blood sugar levels is essential to ensure the well-being of both you and your baby during this period.

Healthy diet: Continue to follow a balanced and nutritious diet postpartum. Focus on consuming a variety of whole, unprocessed foods, and maintain a well-balanced distribution of carbohydrates, proteins, and fats. Adequate nutrition is important for postpartum recovery and managing diabetes.

Physical activity: Engage in regular physical activity as advised by your healthcare provider. Physical activity can help manage blood sugar levels, promote weight loss, boost energy levels, and improve overall well-being. Choose activities that are safe and appropriate for your postpartum recovery phase.

Postpartum mental health support: Pay attention to your mental well-being and seek support if needed. The postpartum period can be challenging, and women with diabetes may have additional concerns. Reach out to your healthcare provider or a mental health professional for support and guidance.

Contraception and family planning: Discuss contraception options with your healthcare provider to determine the most suitable method for you. Proper family planning is important for women with diabetes to ensure a healthy pregnancy and manage their condition effectively in subsequent pregnancies.

Long-term follow-up: Continue regular follow-up visits with your healthcare provider to monitor your diabetes management and address any concerns. Long-term management and monitoring of diabetes are crucial for minimizing the risk of complications and maintaining overall health. Remember to consult with your healthcare provider for personalized guidance and recommendations based on your specific medical history and individual needs.

- ***Importance of continued blood sugar control after delivery***

Continued blood sugar control after delivery is of utmost importance for women with diabetes. Here are some key reasons why maintaining optimal blood sugar levels postpartum is crucial:

Preventing complications: Maintaining good blood sugar control can help prevent both short-term and long-term complications associated with diabetes. These complications include cardiovascular diseases, kidney problems, nerve damage, eye complications, and an increased risk of developing type 2 diabetes later in life.

Promoting postpartum recovery: Adequate blood sugar control supports the body's healing process and postpartum recovery. It helps restore energy levels, promotes tissue repair, and enhances overall well-being.

Managing the risk of recurrence: Gestational diabetes often resolves after delivery. However, women who have had gestational diabetes have a higher risk of developing type 2 diabetes in the future. By maintaining blood sugar control postpartum, women can reduce their risk of developing diabetes in the long term.

Breastfeeding benefits: For women who choose to breastfeed, maintaining stable blood sugar levels is important for milk production and quality. It helps ensure an adequate supply of breast milk and provides optimal nutrition for the baby.

Managing weight and body composition: Effective blood sugar control after delivery can help manage weight and body composition. It supports healthy weight loss postpartum, which is important for overall health and reducing the risk of future complications.

Planning for future pregnancies: Women with diabetes who plan to have more children need to maintain good blood sugar control to optimize their health and minimize risks during future pregnancies. Preconception planning and achieving target blood sugar levels before conception are crucial for a healthy pregnancy.

Overall health and well-being: Stable blood sugar control contributes to improved overall health and well-being. It helps maintain energy levels, regulates mood, reduces the risk of infections, and supports a healthy immune system. Remember, ongoing blood sugar control requires continued monitoring, adherence to a healthy diet, regular physical activity, and close follow-up with healthcare providers. It is essential to work closely with your healthcare team to develop an individualized plan that suits your specific needs and goals for long-term diabetes management.

Conclusion.

In conclusion, diabetes during pregnancy, whether it is gestational diabetes or preexisting diabetes, requires careful management and monitoring to ensure the health and well-being of both the mother and the baby. It is important to work closely with a healthcare team, which may include an obstetrician, endocrinologist or diabetes specialist, registered dietitian, and other healthcare professionals.

Proper management of diabetes during pregnancy involves regular prenatal care, monitoring blood sugar levels, following a healthy diet, engaging in appropriate physical activity, and, if necessary, using medication or insulin therapy. It is crucial to maintain stable blood sugar levels to minimize the risk of complications, such as macrosomia, preterm birth, preeclampsia, and birth defects.

Education and support are essential for women with diabetes during pregnancy. Learning about self-care, blood sugar monitoring, meal planning, and coping strategies can empower women to effectively manage their diabetes and make informed decisions.

After delivery, continued blood sugar control remains important to prevent complications, support postpartum recovery, and manage the risk of recurrence or developing type 2 diabetes. Regular follow-up visits, ongoing blood sugar monitoring, a healthy diet, physical activity, and mental health support are important aspects of postpartum diabetes management.

By effectively managing diabetes during pregnancy and beyond, women can optimize their own health and the health of their baby, reducing the risk of complications and promoting a healthy and successful pregnancy journey.

9 798398 000290